S

By the same Author:
Allergies
Arthritis
Menopause

NUTRITIONAL HEALTH SERIES

STRESS

HOW YOUR DIET CAN HELP

Stephen Terrass

Thorsons

An Imprint of HarperCollins*Publishers*

Dedication

This book is dedicated to Nicola, whose love, understanding, patience, encouragement and valuable input have helped me immeasurably in the writing of the manuscript.

Thorsons
An Imprint of HarperCollins*Publishers*
77–85 Fulham Palace Road,
Hammersmith, London W6 8JB
1160 Battery Street,
San Francisco, California 94111–1213

Published by Thorsons 1994
3 5 7 9 10 8 6 4 2

A catalogue record for this book is
from the British Library

ISBN 0 7225 2986 4

Printed in Great Britain by
HarperCollinsManufacturing, Glasgow

CONTENTS

ACKNOWLEDGEMENTS

The author wishes to thank the following for their valuable support and assistance in this project: Richard Passwater Ph.D. for his inspiration, and for providing the foreword and reviewing the manuscript; editor Sarah Sutton and copy-editor Michele Turney; special thanks to Rand Skolnick, John Steenson, Cheryl Thallon and Leyanne Scharff for their valuable support; and Nibs Laskor for his help and generosity. Most of all, fondest thanks to Nicola Squire and Shirley Terrass for their love and encouragement.

Years ago we learned that nutrition helps us compensate for the ravages of physical stress. Until recently, however, many physicians believed that mental stress was different, and that nutrition had little role in protecting us against it. Now we have verification from sophisticated Magnetic Resonance Images (MRI) which show the effect of mental stress on the brain and other body organs, and how nutrients modify this effect.

We can strive to reduce stress, but there are always deadlines, bills and seemingly insurmountable problems at home or work. While you worry or fume, your body's glands pump out hormones to prepare you to respond. These hormones, in turn, cause other biochemical responses which use up nutrients and 'wear down' your body systems.

Although he may not be able to solve all of your problems, Stephen Terrass can help you protect yourself against the damage that stress can cause. Drawing upon the latest scientific and medical discoveries, he explains how stress affects your body chemistry and what you can do to counteract these harmful reactions, to help restore depleted reserves and to overcome fatigue and exhaustion.

There is no need to let stress cause serious health problems such as heart disease, high blood pressure or frequent headaches. Stephen Terrass recommends nutritional and herbal supplements to help your body chemistry adapt to the effects of constant stress. He presents a programme that makes it easy for you to decide what to do and then gives very clear instructions on how to do it. The complicated biochemistry of stress is presented in an understandable yet thorough style.

Richard A. Passwater, Ph.D.
February 1994

Every day we are exposed to a host of negative influences. These can affect our mood, attitude, general state of mind and perhaps even our health. There is a seemingly endless list of aspects of life that bother us, such as financial problems, family arguments and pressure at work

These factors are all forms of stress. We have become familiar – perhaps too much so – with this term. This means that we tend to accept stress in our lives and do nothing about it, which is one of the main reasons why stress is so damaging to society in general.

It may seem rather naive to suggest that something can be done about stress. While it is often impossible to modify the source of the stress, its effects can be influenced. We are perhaps most familiar with emotional and mental effects, but there are countless other influences, ranging from the mild to the quite severe. Stress is linked to a wide variety of health disorders which are all too prevalent in Western society. One example is cardiovascular disease, the most common cause of death in Britain and the United States.

In spite of our familiarity with its existence, stress is one of the most difficult topics to define in terms of its cause or origin. One problem is that we are all affected differently by stress – what may be stressful for one person may not be so for another. This makes it extremely difficult to approach stress from the standpoint of its source.

There is plenty of helpful information available on how to cope better with circumstances that cause stress. As many stressful situations cannot be avoided, however, it is also vital for people to know what can be done to avoid or minimise the adverse effects stress can have – mental, emotional and, especially, physical. This is the approach taken by this book. It looks into the rather fascinating yet destructive effects that stress can cause, then explores the medically and scientifically proven methods which can be used for reducing such damage and improving one's tolerance to stress in general. This information utilises effective and very safe natural methods including:

- dietary management
- vitamins
- minerals
- herbal medicine

Protecting ourselves from the problems caused by stress is a realistic goal. By utilising the research, it is clear that there are tools to help us to lead a life, not without stress, but perhaps without many of the negative effects that stress can cause. With such information, stress need no longer be an enemy.

CHAPTER 1

What is Stress?

Stress could best be defined as any influence that interrupts or disturbs any aspect of the body's normal functioning. In other words, stress can be caused by just about anything. The generality of this definition reflects the nature of stress itself: it is caused by so many different factors that avoiding it is virtually impossible.

Many people see stress as a side-effect of today's fast-paced lifestyle. As a result, we tend to focus on mental and emotional stress. The truth, however, is that there are many other forms of stress in life.

DIFFERENT TYPES OF STRESS

It is perhaps easier to imagine stress as a pressure or outside force to which our body responds in an unusual way. The part of the body affected depends on the type of outside force. The following descriptions of the different categories of stress will help to outline the various forces that influence us at such a time.

Emotional and Mental Stress

This is the most well-known classification of stress. Our mental and emotional states seem to be so acutely susceptible to react to certain circumstances. Some of these are in the present, some are possible or anticipated occurrences, and some are in the past. Typical forces that exert this type of stress include:

- work problems
- relationship difficulties
- financial worries
- divorce or separation
- being in a hurry
- taking tests or examinations

Such factors seem to have a relatively immediate and adverse effect on us, mentally and emotionally. The initial symptoms of emotional or mental stress vary, but the most common include:

- anger
- anxiety
- worry
- fear
- depression

LEARNED RESPONSE

The outside influence that makes one person emotionally or mentally stressed may have no such effect on another person. Part of the reason for our individual response to such influences lies in our upbringing. From the time we are born, we are conditioned by our circumstances and education, by parents, friends, teachers, religion, etc. As a result, we form an attitude and a way of thinking which may well influence our perception of events from then on. Take as an example a man who becomes upset when his favourite football team loses. The man does not play on the team; he may not even live in the city the team represents. Nevertheless, he has been conditioned to react in what some would say is an irrational manner. This is known as a learned response.

Learned responses can occur in another way as well. They can be more of a habitual reaction which may have been established during childhood. Seemingly irrational fears carried into adulthood, such as a fear of the dark, may be an example of this.

THRESHOLD OF CONFIDENCE

The threshold of a person's confidence often dictates who is likely to be emotionally or mentally stressed by an event. Confidence, or lack of it, is often a semi-rational thing. If, for instance, someone has a phobia about taking tests, this may be due to previous failures, or it may be because he or she is anxious, with good reason, about failing. Often, however, people have a fear of tests even though they have always performed well in them. Take as a good example a man driving a car with manual transmission who stops at the traffic lights on a steep hill. If there is no other car behind his, the driver may easily proceed once the lights change without rolling back or stalling the car. If there is a car behind him, however, he cannot perform what is usually a simple skill for him due to a lack of confidence.

GENERAL STRESS TOLERANCE

A person's general stress tolerance is determined by physiological factors. Regardless of whether stress is being experienced emotionally or mentally, there are always physiological consequences involved as well. This will be discussed throughout the book.

Physical and Environmental Stress

The fact that today's lifestyle is so full of emotional stress often eclipses another form of stress – physical stress. Stress involves *any* influence that disturbs normal functioning, and there are many factors which directly interfere with physical functioning. Some common causes of physical stress include:

- excessive or strenuous exercise
- strenuous physical labour (e.g. lifting and moving too many heavy objects)
- traumatic motion or jolting
- temperature changes (extreme heat or cold)

Physical stress can be minor or more severe depending on the nature of the stressor (something that causes stress). As one's body is more or less able to adjust easily to *gradual* alterations in physical or environmental circumstances, such stress often involves *extremes* of one sort or another: going from extreme heat to extreme cold, for example, or taking up strenuous exercise after a long period of inactivity.

A VICIOUS CIRCLE

Long-term or acute emotional and/or mental stress, invariably leads to a physical manifestation as well. By the same token, extreme physical stress can lead to an emotional and mental effect. This begins a distressing vicious circle whereby it becomes more difficult to extract oneself from stress in general. This is especially a problem when the underlying stress is chronic. Fortunately, regardless of whether the stress is mental, emotional or physical, one is *not* defenceless against its influences. As a matter of fact, not only can we reduce the negative short-term influences of stress, but there are also methods of dealing with the longer-term effects. Such protection, using natural methods, will be discussed later.

CHAPTER 2

The Stress Reaction

If stress did not cause a reaction, people would probably not mind being under stress. After all, stress is just an influence, not a negative experience in itself; it becomes so only when the body has 'processed' the event. Some of the more common reactions to a stressor or stressful event may include the following:

- tension
- muscle stiffness
- perspiration
- hyper-alertness
- altered breathing pattern
- increased heart rate

Sound familiar? These are perhaps the classic initial reactions to stress. But why do we experience them? To the average person they may seem unnecessary and inconvenient. Nobody wants to go into a job interview with sweaty palms, and if you worry about this happening, the reaction is likely to get worse. Nevertheless, the stress reaction, for all its inconvenience, serves a necessary purpose.

The human body has a remarkable system of protective mechanisms for seemingly any occurrence that stresses or runs contrary to the body's intended function. The underlying purpose of every stress reaction is maintaining balance in the body, known as homeostasis. When our body or mind is under stress, we have to function in a different manner in order to deal with it. The body has a system that compensates for this, and its manifestation is the stress reaction itself.

THE ENDOCRINE SYSTEM

Various essential bodily functions are controlled by the endocrine system. These include the reproductive system, growth, metabolism, the immune system, fluid balance, mineral balance, allergic response and stress tolerance. The chemical messengers responsible are called hormones, which are secreted by the glands that make up the endocrine system, such as the adrenal, pituitary and hypothalamus glands.

The Adrenal Glands

The most important glands in terms of stress are the adrenals. Often called the 'anti-stress glands', they are relatively small, and one is located on top of each kidney.

An adrenal gland is made up of two major parts. The outer portion – the adrenal cortex – comprises about

80–90 per cent of the adrenal tissue. The inner portion
– the adrenal medulla – comprises about 10–20 per cent.
Considering their rather small size, the adrenals have
an incredible amount of influence on the human
body. They serve many different purposes in the
body, the most important of which are listed below.

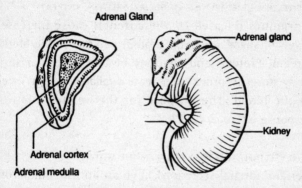

Adrenal Gland

Adrenal gland

Kidney

Adrenal cortex

Adrenal medulla

Fig. 2.1 THE ADRENAL GLANDS

STRESS RESPONSE
(*See pages 12–17.*)

CONTROL OF ALLERGIC RESPONSE
When one reacts in an allergic manner to a particular
substance, the adrenal glands secrete hormones that
dampen the reaction. Drugs comprised of adrenal
hormones are sometimes used to treat severe reactions,
such as asthma.

SEXUAL FUNCTION AND DEVELOPMENT

The adrenals manufacture substances that help regulate sexual functions and characteristics. These include androgens (male sex hormones) and oestrogen (female sex hormone).

CONTROL OF METABOLISM OF SUGAR, PROTEIN, AND FAT

Hormones released by the adrenals cause increased levels of sugar (glucose), protein and fats in the bloodstream. Proteins and fats may be taken from existing body stores in order to increase available energy levels in the blood. The purpose for this relates to stress response (*see pages 12–17*).

REDUCED INFLAMMATORY AND IMMUNE ACTIVITY

Certain adrenal secretions have an anti-inflammatory effect. Adrenal activity can also suppress the immune system.

Adrenal Hormones

Each portion of an adrenal gland, the cortex and the medulla, secretes its own group of hormones. Each type of hormone causes different bodily reactions.

HORMONE	SITE OF RELEASE	FUNCTION
Glucocorticoids (e.g. cortisol, cortisone)	Adrenal cortex	Metabolism of sugar; breakdown of body's fat and protein stores into the blood; involved in suppression of immune system, and of inflammatory and allergic responses.
Mineralocorticoids (e.g. aldosterone)	Adrenal cortex	Retention of sodium in the body; excretion of potassium; involved in mineral regulation.
17-ketosteroids (e.g. androgen sex hormones)	Adrenal cortex	Male characteristics; sex drive
Catecholamines (e.g. adrenaline, noradrenaline)	Adrenal medulla	Increase in heart rate; constriction of blood vessels; altered breathing pattern; promotion of alertness; increase in sweating and metabolic rate; rise in levels of blood sugar and fat; reduction in stores of body fat.

Fig 2.2 THE SOURCES AND FUNCTIONS OF
ADRENAL HORMONES

THE GENERAL ADAPTATION SYNDROME

A stressful situation causes a specific chain reaction in the body. The primary purpose of this reaction is to compensate for the stressor so that the body can regain its normal balance (homeostasis) as soon as possible. Balance can only be accomplished if the body subsequently adapts to the requirements of the event, and the less severe the event, the more easily this adaptation is achieved. This rebalancing process is known as the 'general adaptation syndrome'.

The adrenal hormones are responsible for carrying out this process. The initial shock or onset of the stressful event stimulates the adrenals to begin a chain reaction, which has three separate phases:

Phase 1: Alarm (fight or flight) Response

Phase 1 of the stress reaction was classified and appropriately named 'fight or flight response' by Dr Hans Selye. This alarm stage represents the body's adaptive reaction to danger or threat. Its basic purpose is to prepare the body for immediate action. This raw and primitive skill is still used in today's primarily non-dangerous stressful situations.

Once triggered, the fight or flight response heightens our physical capabilities. A special determination and confidence is manifested as the alarm response essentially blocks out just about everything but the stress at hand. The mechanism of this response is perhaps the most fascinating feature of stress, as the adrenal glands mobilise so many aspects of the body chemistry to accommodate the immediate requirements.

FIGHT OR FLIGHT MECHANISM

This alarm response is triggered by the adrenal medulla, so hormones such as adrenaline and noradrenaline are primarily responsible for the effects (*see figure 2.2*). As we have seen, common initial reactions to stress include symptoms such as hyper-alertness, tension, fast breathing and sweating. Not surprisingly, large quantities of adrenaline and noradrenaline circulating in the bloodstream have considerably similar physiological effects. Common physiological and chemical occurrences of the alarm response are as follows:

- Increased levels of sugar (glucose) and fatty acids are emptied into the bloodstream from the liver and tissues respectively in order to increase available energy supply. This energy can then be used to accommodate the needs of the body to respond to the alarm, and is particularly valuable when immediate and strenuous physical and/or mental action is required. It is used by the brain (causing alertness), the heart, and the working muscles. As these parts of the body take precedence, other areas of the body such as the digestive system will be temporarily deprived of their normal supply of blood.
- The increase in alertness accounts for a higher level

of motivation and determination, among other things.

- Oxygen is also needed for immediate energy. The hormones cause an increased rate of breathing to accommodate this need.
- An increased heart rate allows more blood to be pumped to areas that require substances such as glucose and oxygen to deal with the stress.
- Sweating is stimulated to bring down body temperature and eliminate stress-induced toxins.

Although we tend to consider the early symptoms of stress as negative side-effects, it should now be clear that they are all attributable to a necessary process of physiological compensation.

Phase 2: Resistance Reaction
Stress is not always a short-term phenomenon, especially in modern society. The fight or flight response does not last very long, and if the stress persists past that point, the body must make provisions for longer-term protection. Fortunately the body possesses such a provision. This is the second phase of the general adaptation syndrome, known as the 'resistance reaction'.

When the alarm response wears off, the responsibility of sustaining the body's battle with the stressor switches from the adrenal medulla to the adrenal cortex. The hormones secreted from the cortex – primarily the glucocorticoids and the mineralocorticoids – are mainly responsible for the reaction (*see Figure 2.2*). The two main steps involved in the resistance reaction are as follows:

1 Cortisol (a glucocorticoid) increases blood-sugar levels by causing a breakdown of amino acids from body tissues into sources of useable sugar. As with the effect on glucose in the alarm response, this aids in increasing the availability of energy so that the body can continue to work at a higher rate under stress.
2 By helping the body retain sodium and excrete potassium, aldosterone (a mineralocorticoid) maintains a higher level of blood pressure during prolonged periods of stress. Although we tend to think of increased blood pressure as negative, there are times when it must be higher in order to allow the body to carry out certain circulatory tasks relevant to stress reactions.

The resistance reaction is unquestionably a necessary phase in allowing the body to adapt to more prolonged stress. For many people, the prolonged variety is very common indeed. As the body is equipped with such a mechanism, it might reasonably be assumed that stress is not harmful, no matter how often we are affected by it. Unfortunately, this is not the case. The stress itself may be dealt with time and time again, but serious problems can occur as a result of Phases 1 and (especially) 2 of the general adaptation syndrome.

PROBLEMS WITH REPEATED STRESS

Few things are as emotionally debilitating as chronic stress. If the source of stress is the office, for example, sufferers may come to dread each day at work. If the stress is home-based, sufferers may become work aholics in order to avoid family life. The list goes on and on. The end result of such a situation is often depression, despair and a feeling of helplessness. Such emotions are counterproductive and, do not give sufferers what they require – the energy and confidence to try to improve their situation. Emotional and/or mental stress is, therefore, a self-perpetuating process.

Chronic physical stressors can produce a degree of mental stress as few people will look forward to a situation where their body will be subjected to excessive punishment or trauma. If the physical stressor is chronic, it can also cause emotional stress, which starts another unfortunate cycle of problems.

The higher levels of circulating adrenal hormones, especially corticosteroids, can themselves also be damaging to physical health. As corticosteroids control so many aspects of the body's processes, any imbalance in their normal amount can affect various functions. Catecholamines can also produce problems (*see Chapter Three, pages 26–27*).

Phase 3: Exhaustion
The human body was not designed for constant stress,

and the longer we are exposed to it, the less able the body is to deal with it. If the resistance reaction is pushed beyond its limits, the body hits the final stage of the general adaptation syndrome – 'exhaustion'.

Most of us think of exhaustion as a powerful sense of physical or mental fatigue. Although this is certainly one of the ways in which exhaustion can be experienced, it can also be linked more specifically to certain, perhaps many, parts of the body, which cease to be able to function at their intended capacity, and perhaps just 'give out' or collapse.

LIMITED SUPPLY OF HORMONES

The activity of the adrenal hormones not only accounts for stress reactions, but also for stress tolerance. Unfortunately, we do not have an unending supply of adrenal hormones. These must be manufactured by the body in adequate quantities to compensate for the draining of the supply during stress.

The adrenal hormones are made 'from scratch', and the body uses certain food nutrients as ingredients in the recipe. If the ingredients are in too short a supply, or if the stress requirements use the hormones faster than they can be manufactured, then the body can no longer deal with further stress. As adrenal hormones are responsible for all the other necessary functions carried out by the adrenal glands in addition to stress reactions, any lack of supply means that those processes do not happen as they should either. This is where collapse or dysfunction of various body systems can occur.

The phenomenon of adrenal 'uselessness' due to lack of hormones is often called 'adrenal exhaustion'. When the adrenals become exhausted, stress tolerance decreases, and the supply of blood sugar is depleted as well. The latter is particularly damaging. When stress is being dealt with, the adrenal hormones mobilise various supplies of energy to increase levels of blood sugar, which allows the brain, heart and muscles to work at a higher rate (*see pages 12–14*). If the supply of adrenal hormones is exhausted, then the opposite occurs. The blood-sugar level falls perpetually low (hypoglycaemia), which causes the brain, heart, muscles and all the other cells in the body to be negatively affected.

BREAKDOWN OF BODY SYSTEMS

It is difficult to say which parts of the body are most susceptible to damage from adrenal exhaustion. It presumably depends on the strength of the various parts prior to the event. The adrenal glands themselves become extremely weak, partly due to being overworked, and partly due to the short supply of energy from the blood (healthy adrenals receive an extremely high volume of blood per day for their size). The cardiovascular system also takes a great pounding from the problem. This is partly due to the potentially damaging effect of adrenal hormones on the system through factors such as increased blood pressure and constriction of blood vessels, and partly due to the fact that the heart is a quick recipient of the energy mobilised by the adrenal hormones under stress.

INITIAL SYMPTOMS

Before a severe breakdown of major body systems takes place, adrenal exhaustion itself can cause more nagging symptoms. The first noticeable reaction may be a reduced ability to adjust to a stressful situation. This could manifest during both emotional/mental stress, as well as physical stress.

In the case of emotional stress, the decreased stress tolerance is enough to make a mild stress situation intolerable. When mental stress is involved, you have the combination of both the reduced stress tolerance, as well as the reduced energy going to the brain due to a lack of blood sugar. This may cause lack of mental alertness, mental fatigue in general, depression and dizziness. When one is under physical stress, reduced stress tolerance and reduced sugar to the working muscles can make normal physical exertion difficult to accomplish. General physical fatigue becomes chronic.

In order to try and compensate for the low blood sugar (hypoglycaemia) caused by the adrenal hormone deficiency, the body will often crave sugar and refined carbohydrates. This craving creates problems of its own (*see page 56–59*).

Summary of General Adaptation Syndrome

PHASE 1: ALARM RESPONSE

- 'fight or flight' response
- preparation of the body for action
- increased energy from blood to brain, heart, working muscles
- regulated by catecholamines (adrenaline, noradrenaline)

PHASE 2: RESISTANCE REACTION

- maintenance of stress response after alarm reaction wears off
- creation of energy from amino acids to sustain stress reaction
- regulated by corticosteroids (cortisol, cortisone, aldosterone)

PHASE 3: EXHAUSTION

- weakened supply of adrenal hormones
- general mental and physical fatigue and hypo-glycaemia
- breakdown of function of weakened body systems

From personal experience it is easy to recognise each stage of the general adaptation syndrome by the associated physiological changes. We have all experienced the jolt of energy and tension, the sweaty palms, the hyper-alertness, the increased breathing and heart rate that accompany the fight or flight response. You are also likely to have remained in a state of stress long after the initial rush is over (phase 2).

To what extent you might have experienced the effects of the third phase depends on many factors. A preliminary version is, however, manifested in the minor fatigue one experiences after a prolonged period of stress. In the earlier stages, or provided prolonged stress is not a regular feature of your life, your body (and hormone supply) can replenish itself.

As you begin to understand the rather fascinating dynamics of stress within the body, it may help you to realise that there is more to stress than you ever imagined. The next chapter takes this even further, and explains the more long-term effects that stress can have on the body. Chapter Three will also clarify the fact that chronic stress is something which does need to be addressed in order to maintain optimal physical as well as mental and emotional health.

CHAPTER 3

The Effects of Stress on Health

Although stress can have an adverse affect on almost every part of the body, certain reactions caused by stress tend to pinpoint specific areas. Research has revealed which parts of the body are most likely to be harmed and what form such damage takes. It is important to remember that it is the stress reaction, rather than the stressor itself, that generally causes problems. You may find it useful to refer back to Figure 2.2 'The sources and functions of adrenal hormones' throughout this chapter (*see page 11*)

STRESS AND CARDIOVASCULAR DISEASE

The term 'cardiovascular' refers to the heart, and to the body's system of blood vessels. Cardiovascular disease is possibly the most serious health problem that can be linked to stress. In Britain and the United States, this disease is the most common cause of death. The prevalence of cardiovascular disease in these countries is usually linked to dietary problems, and to habits such as smoking. While these may be the primary measurable factors, stress can also play a disturbing role.

Some of the more common disorders or diseases of the cardiovascular system include:

- high blood pressure (hypertension)
- atherosclerosis (hardening of the arteries)
- heart attack
- congestive heart failure
- stroke (a cerebrovascular disease)
- angina

The presence of any of the following circumstances in the cardiovascular system increases the risk of heart disease:

1 a tendency towards weakness of, or injury to, the blood vessels
2 weakness of the heart muscle
3 an increased development of blood plaque (a formation of substances which clog the blood vessel and restrict circulation)

High Blood Pressure

Blood vessels are tubes that transport blood throughout the body. Arteries are blood vessels that carry blood pumped from the heart to the different parts of the body. When the blood vessel is able to open more widely (dilate), more blood can flow freely with less pressure on the vessel walls. If the blood vessel is tapered in a particular area (constricted), then the blood flow reduces and exerts more pressure on the walls of the vessel.

When you use your thumb to partially block the flow of water through a garden hose, the water flow through that space becomes more turbulent. If the wall of the hose is very thin and weak, the water begins to cause a swelling, further weakening the walls in the site of the constriction. If you equate this story to the blood vessels, it is not difficult to imagine some of the problems that may occur if the blood flow is restricted in a particular area.

POTASSIUM, SODIUM AND BLOOD PRESSURE

Blood pressure (pressure exerted against the walls of blood vessels) is controlled by several factors. Two minerals, potassium and sodium (often called electrolytes), make up a large part of the equation.

Sodium is linked to:

1 constriction of the blood vessels
2 an increase in volume of plasma (the fluid of the blood)

Both these factors result in an increased pressure on the vessels walls, or higher blood pressure.

Potassium, on the other hand, is linked with vessel dilation (vasodilation) and the relaxation of the muscles of the blood vessels. This encourages the easier flow of blood through the vessels, and also causes a reduction in the retention of sodium and fluid. Both factors should lower the blood pressure.

Sodium and potassium are in constant competition with one another. If sodium levels are too high, potassium must be increased to counterbalance sodium's effects, and vice versa. So what does this have to do with stress?

ADRENAL HORMONES AND BLOOD PRESSURE

Several hormones secreted by the adrenals (*see page 11*) have a direct effect on blood pressure. Adrenaline, secreted in the alarm phase of the stress event, is a blood vessel constricting agent (vasoconstrictor). Cortisol and aldosterone cause potassium to be excreted and sodium to be retained (aldosterone is much more potent in this effect). All three hormones cause blood pressure to increase.

If the stress is short-lived, or at least not a regular feature of the sufferer's life, this rise in blood pressure should correct itself and not cause any serious or lasting harm to the body. The problem exists when the stress is chronic. A frequent or perpetual state of high blood pressure may indeed have long-term consequences.

High blood pressure, or hypertension, is a primary risk factor in death from heart disease. It is not only linked to potassium/sodium balance, but may also be a warning sign of blocked arteries. Nevertheless, reduction in chronic stress – or rather a reduction in chronic stress reactions – may lead to a considerably lower risk of high blood pressure and heart disease.

Atherosclerosis

Atherosclerosis, or hardening of the arteries, is another cardiovascular complication that can be linked to stress. By far the major determining factor in the risk of dying of heart disease, atherosclerosis is characterised by the development of blood plaque in the arteries, which progressively narrows the pathway through which the blood can flow. Eventually the opening can become blocked, which can result in high blood pressure, angina, stroke, heart attack, etc. Ultimately, and for a shockingly high percentage of the population in Britain and the United States, this will lead to premature death from heart failure or attack.

ARTERIAL INJURY

Although there are many theories on what causes the development of atherosclerosis, one of the most widely accepted is that of arterial injury. If the wall of an artery is injured, several substances are diverted to the lesion during the healing process. It appears that other substances, such as cholesterol, get caught up in the injured tissue and are deposited there. This leads to an accumulation of cholesterol deposits, the fibrous tissue involved in healing the area, white blood cells, smooth muscle cells and other substances. Eventually a clot begins to form; and if it continues to grow, it can block the artery. Ironically, then, it is the healing process itself that can lead to the formation of a clot, but this should be seen in context – severe arterial injury is not a normal occurrence. In a society with a better diet, including a lower intake of oxidised fats, and more suitable blood-pressure levels, there would be far less likelihood of such problems.

The cause of the initial arterial injury depends on the person. It has been suggested, however, that increased blood pressure may well be a common cause. If potassium levels are inadequate to maintain proper flexibility of the vessel walls, and to prevent excessive vasoconstriction, then there could be problems. Weakening of the blood vessel wall from the 'stress' of the increased blood pressure, combined with the turbulent flow through the constricted pathway may cause eventual injury to the wall.

Stress can be implicated in such a development, due to its ability to increase blood pressure. When the injury, and thus the blockage, begins to occur, the blood pressure will increase further still, thereby producing a rather negative chain reaction.

As you can see, the impact of stress on the cardiovascular system can be disastrous. Any manifestation of cardiovascular disease is capable of being at least partially caused, and certainly made worse, by stress.

STRESS AND THE IMMUNE SYSTEM

The immune system protects us from infection. It fights foreign invaders (such as viruses and harmful bacteria) and cancer. The immune system is made up of many components. The most relevant to stress are the white blood cells and the thymus gland.

White Blood Cells

There are several types of white blood cells:

T-CELLS

T-cells are produced in the thymus gland, and come in three different forms:

- T-helper cells, which increase immune activity
- T-suppressor cells, which decrease immune activity
- cytotoxic T-cells, which attack infected cells

T-cells also manufacture interferon, a vital immune substance.

B-CELLS

Produced in the bone marrow, B-cells manufacture antibodies that bond to invaders. This starts up a chain reaction during which the invader is destroyed by other white blood cells.

OTHER WHITE BLOOD CELLS

These include:

- neutrophils, which destroy cancer cells and bacteria
- natural killer cells (NK), which kill cells infected with viruses or cancer

Thymus Gland

The thymus gland has two principal functions:

1 manufacturing T-cells (essential for regulating immunity)
2 manufacturing immune-related hormones

Impaired Immune Function

Due to its primary function in the body, the immune system has incredible scope – when it is working properly. If it is not working as it should, for whatever reason, the implications can be disastrous.

The purpose of a stress reaction is to mobilise resources to the parts of the body that need to deal with the stress (*see pages 12–14*), mainly the brain, heart and working muscles (such as the legs when a person has to run very quickly). As a result, all the bodily systems that are deemed unnecessary in fighting the stress are temporarily deprived of resources, including the immune system.

The thymus, as mentioned above, plays a huge and essential role in the function of the immune system. Besides making the white blood cells responsible for regulating a multitude of different immune responses, the thymus also releases hormones that are potent immune stimulants – substances that trigger or directly carry out the destruction of invaders, cancer development etc. Any harm to the function of the thymus causes untold damage to immunity in general, and stress does cause harm to the thymus. Adrenal hormones, such as cortisol and cortisone, actually cause the thymus gland to shrink. In cases of chronic stress, this effect can be substantial, and the implications quite severe.

Stress also affects the white blood cells. Corticosteroids, the hormones secreted by the adrenal cortex (such as cortisol), are known to reduce the activity of certain white blood cells that are absolutely essential for resistance to infection and other vital processes of the immune system. In certain diseases, such as rheumatoid arthritis and ulcerative colitis, corticosteroids are sometimes given as a drug *deliberately* to suppress the immune system in this way. These drugs do not cure the condition, however, and are notorious for their harmful side-effects.

Secreted during stress, the corticosteroids will generally reduce the resistance to infection as well as to the development of cancer cells. There are countless varieties of infection able to infiltrate your system, but some of the more common occurrences relate to colds, influenza and the herpes class viruses (e.g. cold sores). Provided the stress is temporary, this reduced resistance will not last long. If the stress is chronic, however, then the immune system may spend much of its time being underactive. This phenomenon also helps to explain why we are more likely to catch a cold, for example, when our stress levels are at their highest.

CANCER

There is another suggested link between stress and cancer. As well as the decrease in the activity of certain cancer cell-destroying white blood cells, the effect of adrenal hormones on the thymus is particularly disturbing.

As the thymus is the producer of the immune-regulating T-cells and immune hormones, any damage through shrinkage increases the risk of cancer cells developing. The T-cells also produce the vital immune substance interferon in response to cancer-cell development. If the T-cells are impeded in their function or are present in abnormally low quantities due to thymus shrinkage, then cancer protection may be reduced from this angle as well.

One should not assume that regular stress will lead to cancer. It is, however, important not to take chronic stress too lightly. The stressors in one's life may always be a factor, but the ways in which the body deals with it can be improved. Such methods will be discussed in Chapter Six.

STRESS AND INFLAMMATORY CONDITIONS

As mentioned earlier, corticosteroids have an anti-inflammatory effect. If a person is under chronic stress to the point where the adrenals become exhausted of their strength and hormonal supply, then the ability of the body to fight inflammation is reduced.

Rheumatoid Arthritis

Stress may be in factor in rheumatoid arthritis. In this type of arthritis, the immune system mistakenly attacks the joints, leading to substantial swelling, redness and heat in the affected joints (inflammation). If the sufferer's natural supply of corticosteroids is lacking, then the inflammatory symptoms and associated problems of such diseases may be worse than they would otherwise have been.

Auto-immune Diseases

As with rheumatoid arthritis, other diseases are caused by the immune system attacking body tissues rather than their intended enemies, such as viruses, cancer cells and bacteria. The more well-known of these auto-immune diseases include multiple sclerosis (MS), ulcerative colitis, rheumatoid arthritis and lupus erythematosus.

   Although there can be many different factors that cause the white blood cells to mistakenly attack the body, a disorder of the activity of thymus-derived T-helper and suppressor cells may be involved. If the thymus is damaged by stress, it is anybody's guess as to what the activity of the T-helper and T-suppressor cells is going to be.

STRESS AND ALLERGIES

Allergic reactions are a result of inflammation in various tissues. Like inflammatory conditions, they are suppressed by corticosteroids, but also by adrenaline. In cases of adrenal exhaustion, the action of the adrenaline would be reduced. As a result, conditions related to allergies may well be manifested more readily when one is under chronic stress.

Asthma

Perhaps one of the better examples of this phenomenon is asthma. This condition, which is brought about by constriction of the breathing passages, is often connected to allergies. Inflammation can occur in the small airways (bronchioles) in the lungs which narrows the opening, thus restricting normal breathing. A reduction in anti-inflammatory and anti-allergic adrenal hormones on demand may create a higher likelihood of an asthma attack. Drugs containing these hormones are often used in asthma control.

STRESS AND DIABETES

Diabetes is a condition brought about by an inability to metabolise sugar correctly, leading to excessively high levels of sugar in the blood. The responsibility for such metabolism falls on the hormone insulin which is secreted by the pancreas.

In today's society, diabetes represents one of the more distressing health disorders. If it reaches a certain point without being controlled, it can be fatal. In spite of the current diagnostic measures, which can also be performed at home, and the availability of controlling drugs, diabetes is quickly growing, rather than reducing, in incidence. The only conclusion that can be drawn from this is that Western society perpetuates the risk of diabetes.

The vast majority of diabetics fall under the category 'type 2'. Such a diabetic is not unable to manufacture insulin, but the insulin is not able to do its job properly. Once insulin enters the bloodstream it must successfully attach itself to an insulin receptor on the surface of the cell. In this way it can metabolise the sugar, leading to a consequent drop in blood-sugar levels. In type 2 diabetics, some factor interrupts this process (known as insulin sensitivity).

Adrenal Hormones and Blood Sugar

As previously discussed, the release of adrenal

hormones under stress can have substantial effects on blood-sugar levels (*see page 19*). Adrenaline causes glucose stored in the liver to be dumped into the bloodstream. Corticosteroids, such as cortisol, not only increase blood sugar by breaking down protein, they also reduce the metabolism of glucose by the cells. Very large amounts of cortisol decrease insulin sensitivity.

As with high blood pressure, if the high blood-sugar levels (and decreased insulin sensitivity) are not chronic, then there should be no long-term problems. In chronic stress, however, it is clear that a diabetic tendency can easily emerge, especially if the person carries other common traits of the type 2 diabetic, such as obesity and/or a high sugar consumption.

MISCELLANEOUS HEALTH PROBLEMS

Headaches
Many different aspects of stress can produce headaches. The adverse long-term effect of stress on the nervous system may make a sufferer more sensitive to pain in the first place. The muscle tension experienced in the neck and shoulders may make matters worse. Another problem arises due to the constricting effect of adrenal hormones on blood circulation. Although the circulation to the brain increases in the initial phase of stress, the long-term effect of chronic stress on circulation in

general may be negative. This may eventually adversely affect blood flow to the brain and lead to headaches.

Premenstrual Tension (PMT)

In addition to the effect of stress on the nerves in general, certain premenstrual symptoms may be worsened by stress. Many sufferers of PMT have higher than usual levels of the adrenal hormone aldosterone. This may account for some or much of the problem of excessive fluid weight gain, general fluid retention, breast tenderness and abdominal bloating. Further aldosterone release from general stress will make such matters worse.

Depression

The psychological effects of chronic stress often lead to depression, but physiological factors can also contribute to this condition. Adrenaline and noradrenaline are not only adrenal hormones, but also chemical messengers in the brain. Deficiencies in noradrenaline have been linked to depression in some individuals. If circulating noradrenaline levels are low, perhaps as a result of adrenal exhaustion, then depression may occur.

Digestive and Intestinal Disturbances

Many problems of the digestive tract, such as indigestion, gas, heartburn and irritable bowel, are linked with stress. Although irritable bowel syndrome (IBS) is often thought to be caused by stress, research shows that stress is probably not the initial cause, although it does make the problem worse.

The nerves in the intestines receive hormonal messages from the brain that tell the intestinal muscles to stretch and contract, for example. Any imbalance in the timing or quantity (too much or too little) of the release of such hormones can cause alterations in intestinal function, such as spasms, diarrhoea and constipation. Along with its adverse effect on the nerves, stress causes the digestive system more or less to shut down for a time. This may be a major factor in the above digestive and intestinal problems.

ULCERS

The connection between stress and peptic ulcers has not been proven beyond doubt in research. Some people's ulcers are probably linked to stress, but others may be due to different factors.

Nevertheless, it is clear from the research that stress can definitely be an major factor in causing many health problems and making others worse. The most important consideration, however, is not the number of stressors a sufferer is subjected to, but how the body deals with the stress.

Coping with stress from a psychological standpoint can be very difficult. The factors involved are heavily influenced by personality type, upbringing, environment, religious beliefs, etc. Our perception of events, and any habitual reactions to types of events, will figure in this equation as well. From a physiological angle, the picture is fortunately far clearer, and there are certain rules that almost anyone can follow to increase their stress tolerance successfully. The following chapters will give you the necessary information to help you do this.

CHAPTER 4

Analysing Your Stress and Stress Tolerance

An important step in the initial process of tackling stress, and the effects that it has on body and mind, is to look at the stresses in your life. It can be very helpful to assess stress in many different ways and for many reasons. There are three main steps in this process:

1. IDENTIFYING THE SOURCES OF THE PROBLEM

If any of the common sources of stress to which you are exposed can feasibly be avoided, then it may be wise to do so. Although this advice may seem elementary, someone suffering from stress from many different angles or sources may become oblivious to the stress created by some of them.

2. SEPARATING STRESSORS INTO RELEVANT CATEGORIES

Categorising the stressors in your life can help you compensate for your stress. Such categories include emotional stressors, mental stressors, and physical and environmental stressors *(see Chapter Five)* . It may also be helpful to categorise your stresses as either under your control or choosing, or out of your control. Identifying sources out of your control, such as the actions or words of others, means that you can concentrate on manipulating your reactions in order to cope with the stress – practising deep breathing, for example.

3. ASSESSING THE FREQUENCY OF EXPOSURE TO STRESSORS

Looking at the frequency and/or volume of stressors can help us to assess the likelihood of impending physical problems, such as over-taxed adrenals. The necessary steps can then be taken to bolster the body's anti-stress network *(see Chapter Five)* .

RATING THE EFFECT OF LIFE CHANGES OR EVENTS

The following list of life events and changes was devised by Thomas Holmes and Richard Rahe, and published in the *Journal of Psychosomatic Research* (no. 11) in 1967. It still stands as a useful tool in helping to assess the possible stress implications of various life changes and events. Use it to give you a better idea of just how stressed you are.

Stress Ratings of Life Changes and Events

The following list is meant to give you an idea of how stressful certain life events are in relation to others. The higher the score, the more stressful the event.

1   death of spouse 100
2   divorce 73
3   marital separation 65
4   jail sentence 63
5   death of close family member 63
6   injury or illness 53
7   marriage 50
8   fired from job 47
9   marital reconciliation 45
10   retirement 45
11   health problem of family member 44
12   pregnancy 40
13   sex problems 39
14   new family member 39
15   business changes or adjustment 39
16   change in financial situation 38
17   death of close friend 37
18   change in line of work 36
19   change in amount of arguments with spouse 35
20   large mortgage 31
21   loan or mortgage foreclosure 30
22   change in work duties 29
23   child leaving home 29
24   problems with in-laws 29

25   major personal achievement 28
26   wife starts or stops work 26
27   beginning or ending school 26
28   change in living conditions 25
29   change in personal habits 24
30   problems with boss 23
31   change in work hours or condition 20
32   moving residence 20
33   change in school 20
34   change in recreation 19
35   change in church activities 19
36   change in social activities 18
37   taking out small mortgage 17
38   change in sleep habits 16
39   change in number of family get-togethers 15
40   changes in eating habits 15
41   holiday/vacation 13
42   Christmas 12
43   minor violation of the law 11

Further Stress-assessment Questions

Aside from the above chart, it is important to look at other, more general, factors in your life that can be a source of stress. These are just a few of the questions you may want to ask yourself in order to get a better idea of your situation.

• Are you frequently in a hurry/always running late?
• Do you have more appointments in a day than can be achieved in a relaxed manner?

- Are you constantly fighting traffic/crowds?
- Do you live in a highly polluted environment (e.g. air pollution, noise)?
- Do you have a mentally/emotionally strenuous job?
- Do you have a physically strenuous job?
- Do you over-exert yourself in physical exercise?
- Do you lack physical activity?
- Are you constantly fighting infections?
- Are you exposed to extremes or severe fluctuation in temperature, climate, etc.?
- Are you frequently deprived of sleep?

SIGNS AND SYMPTOMS OF EXCESSIVE STRESS

We looked earlier at some of the more common symptoms of stress reactions (see pages 12–14). It is also important not to ignore various signs and symptoms which could be telling you that your body is under *excessive* stress and losing its ability to tolerate stress (perhaps through adrenal weakness or exhaustion). The following list concentrates more on the physiological, rather than psychological, symptoms:

- nervousness/irritability/anxiety
- insomnia
- chronic indigestion, gas or bloating after meals
- chronic headaches
- recently discovered allergies

- loss of sex drive
- shortness of breath
- heart palpitations
- high blood pressure
- chronic infections
- chronic fatigue
- chronic constipation and/or diarrhoea
- excessive cravings for sugar, caffeine, tobacco or alcohol
- depression
- lack of mental alertness
- inability to concentrate
- dizziness
- muscle spasms or cramps
- skin rashes, eruptions or irritations
- lack of appetite
- lack of tolerance for physical activity

These are just some of the warning signs that may be telling you that your combined stresses have reached a level your body cannot tolerate. Although it would perhaps be preferable, this does *not* mean that you have no choice but to lessen the quantity of stresses in order to allow your body to tolerate the load. If you cannot eliminate the stresses, then you can strengthen the body's ability to cope.

It may be helpful to run down the above list and mark each symptom or sign that applies to you. Any one of these could be caused by stress, particularly by stress levels in excess of your body's tolerance. If a few, or perhaps many, currently apply to you, and you know that chronic stress certainly is a factor in your life, then it may be worth while to address the anti-stress information in Chapters Five and Six. Even if you suffer from none of the above signs yet know that your levels of stress are chronic, the information in these chapters may help to reduce the risks of such problems later on.

Going through all of the steps in this chapter may give you a very practical stress profile. This is *not*, however, a substitute for qualified psychological counselling where required.

CHAPTER 5

Diet and Stress

Once you are satisfied that you have gone through any necessary evaluation of your situation, the next step is to decide what to do about it. Fortunately, there is something which can be done about stress. This book cannot tell you how to remove stress from your life, but it does outline methods that may:

1 increase your tolerance for stress
2 reduce the adverse physiological effects of stress
3 reduce the chance of, or the effects of, adrenal weakness or exhaustion
4 help you maintain a better state of health

The advice given in this chapter and Chapter Six is based on published scientific and medical research and utilises strictly *natural* methods of prevention and/or treatment. These methods have been widely proven to be effective and safe in treating not only stress-related effects but also conditions closely linked with stress, such as cardiovascular disease and immune disorders. Although these next chapters concentrate more on general methods of increasing stress-protection and tolerance, there will also be some references to dealing with specific problems.

This chapter looks at how our diet can substantially influence our tolerance for, and response to stress, both positively and negatively. Use this information to assess whether your diet is helping or hurting your tolerance to the effects of stress.

NEGATIVE DIETARY ELEMENTS

From research into the effects of various substances on the human body, it is possible to draw up some general rules which should apply to almost anyone. Firstly, it is important to know which elements of your diet could be having a negative effect on your stress tolerance.

Caffeine

Caffeine is a stimulant found in many commonly consumed foods and drinks, including coffee, tea, chocolate, and soft drinks such as colas. It is also found in some painkillers.

Although it is a drug, the use of caffeine is not legally restricted. In Western society, it is socially acceptable to consume fairly large amounts of the substance. As a result, caffeine is not generally viewed as particularly harmful. This is misleading. The truth is that caffeine is not harmless when consumed in the quantities that many do each day, and it is particularly unhelpful to people suffering from chronic stress. Furthermore, this is not just a general point about dietary vices; it is a research-proven point which should be clearly understood, especially by highly stressed individuals.

CAFFEINE AND THE ADRENALS

Beverages that contain caffeine, such as coffee, have been shown to cause a rise in the release of adrenaline. This helps to explain certain symptoms that have been linked with excessive caffeine consumption, such as nervous tension, irritability and insomnia.

Besides these overt symptoms, the adverse effects of caffeine on the adrenal glands may be more far-reaching. One of the problems caused by adrenaline release as the result of chronic stress is a possible exhaustion of the supply (*see pages 16–19*). This may happen faster if the sufferer is consuming agents that further stimulate such a process when the body does not really require it.

CAFFEINE AND CARDIOVASCULAR DISEASE

There is also a connection between caffeine intake and high blood pressure, although it is still relatively unclear. Despite the fact that some research suggests the body will adjust in time to any increase in blood pressure, when the effect of caffeine is combined with the adverse effect of stress, the caffeine would be well worth avoiding, or at least reducing.

Several studies have proven a significant link

between coffee consumption and high cholesterol levels. This increase is particularly noticeable in the levels of LDL cholesterol, which is the negative type. It appears that drinking five or more cups of coffee per day is especially harmful, although fewer can also cause increases. Research has also revealed that tea does not create the same problems. This may be because tea contains less caffeine than coffee, a supposition backed up by the finding that decaffeinated coffee does not cause increases in cholesterol levels.

TEA, COFFEE AND NUTRIENTS

Tea and coffee have also been found to have some negative effects on nutrient utilisation. They are known to reduce the absorption of the minerals zinc and iron. Zinc plays a particularly important role in stress protection, as it is involved in the production of adrenal hormones. Research has also shown that a large amount of the mineral calcium is lost in the urine after caffeine ingestion. Calcium plays an important part in the function of the nervous system and in controlling high blood pressure. Caffeine is also classified as a diuretic, which means that it causes the rapid elimination of fluid. Diuretics are notorious for their unbalancing effects on many important nutrients, including ones involved in the nervous system and stress protection.

Alcohol

Another commonly consumed drug, alcohol is in a

class of its own as far as destructive effects are concerned. Although the list of these effects is far too long to cover completely here, there are a few areas of particular importance that should be noted.

ALCOHOL AND THE ADRENALS

Like caffeine, alcohol stimulates the secretion of adrenaline, producing the same associated problems as caffeine (*see above*).

ALCOHOL AND NUTRIENTS

Alcohol can have a negative effect of a vast range of nutrients, including many that are vital to the healthy functioning of the adrenal glands and the nervous, immune and cardiovascular systems. It could safely be said that excessive alcohol could be a problem to more or less the entire body, and not least to stress tolerance and adrenal health.

ALCOHOL AND THE LIVER

The well-known fact that alcohol harms liver function can have many different implications, but the one most relevant to stress is the possible impairment of detoxification. The liver is responsible for eliminating toxic substances from the body. These include hormones such as cortisol and aldosterone, which are released in large amounts during stress. Such detoxification is a necessary process, and if the liver is compromised in any way – such as through excess alcohol – then this will not be so efficiently carried out. The higher the level of such hormones in circulation, the more important this task is.

Smoking

We are all aware of many of the hazards of smoking, particularly in terms of cancer and heart disease. The damage that smoking can do in these areas is mostly attributable to the effect of the smoke itself. Where stress is concerned, however, nicotine is the main problem.

NICOTINE AND ADRENAL FUNCTION

Nicotine is a stimulant drug, and is thus responsible for the most attractive attributes of cigarette smoking, such as increased alertness and stress tolerance. If nicotine increases stress tolerance in smokers, you may justifiably wonder why smoking is listed under negative effects.

One of the most important things to remember is that stress tolerance is dictated, to a great extent, by the levels of circulating adrenal hormones. Nicotine is yet another example of a drug that increases adrenaline secretion. When one smokes, the adrenaline increases, thereby easing the stress effect.

Although smokers often say that nicotine improves their stress tolerance, it has been found to have a very different effect on non-smokers who may find that the excessive adrenaline levels exacerbate stress symptoms such as tension and anxiety. From this information, one could make the logical assumption that smokers become dependent on nicotine to stimulate stress-relieving adrenaline, and thus cannot secrete it so efficiently themselves if not smoking. This is not so far-fetched when you consider the fact that regular smokers will become addicted to nicotine, and that smokers have such abnormally low levels of stress tolerance when they initially try to quit.

Nicotine is a perfect example of a drug that can lead very quickly to adrenal sluggishness, which is manifested through this dependency during stress. In some people, this may eventually result in hormone levels becoming exhausted.

SMOKING AND NUTRIENTS

Smoking has an adverse effect on the body's supply of necessary nutrients, which can be damaging to adrenal health. The body is quickly drained of its supplies of Vitamin C, which is vital for adrenal hormones to function healthily. Other nutrients are likely to be negatively affected, especially certain B-vitamins.

OTHER PROBLEMS

Smoking may also worsen other risk factors associated with stress including:

- heart disease (high blood pressure, atherosclerosis)
- cancer
- poor digestion
- weakened immunity

Due to smokers' apparent dependency on nicotine for adequate stress-hormone release, those who wish to quit might turn to other stimulants, such as caffeine or sugar, to compensate. Although this may appear to be trading one harmful vice for another, avoiding the damaging effect of the smoke itself on the lungs and cardiovascular system would be helpful. Nevertheless, a proper stress-protection approach, such as that outlined in Chapter Six, may improve stress tolerance, and eventually reduce the need to rely on such stimulants at all.

Sugar
Sugar is a rather confusing subject. On one hand, it represents a major source of energy; yet on the other hand, it can be quite harmful if consumed in excessive amounts and/or in the wrong form.

Dietary sources of sugar are known as carbohydrates. These can be divided into two categories – simple and complex – both of which have somewhat different effects on the body. Simple carbohydrates are sources of dietary sugars which enter the bloodstream quickly and provide an almost instant supply of energy. Complex carbohydrates have to be broken down into simple sugars before they can be used in this way.

The fact that simple carbohydrates are a more immediate energy source may seem like a positive attribute. From the standpoint of health, however, the opposite is often true. Although the body needs sugars, amounts in excess of its immediate energy requirements can create problems. Some of the excess may be stored as fat, an excess of which can lead to obesity, vascular disorders etc.; it may cause blood-sugar imbalances; and it can weaken the cardiovascular and immune systems. Such problems are more likely to occur with refined forms of sugar, such as common white sugar (sucrose).

Some forms of simple carbohydrate sources include:

- white and brown sugar
- honey
- fruits and fruit juices
- glucose
- fructose

Although fruits represent a source of simple carbohydrates, they do not generally cause the same problems as the elements listed above. This is true for the following reasons:

1 fruits contain a high amount of water which helps dilute the contained sugar concentration
2 fruits often contain large amounts of certain types of dietary fibre which may even help to balance blood sugar levels
3 fruits contain nutrients and other valuable substances which may aid in sugar metabolism and help reduce the adverse effects of sugar in general

Bear in mind that it is much better to eat fruit rather than drink fruit juices, as the juice will not contain the fibre and may well be doctored with additives, especially sugar.

SUGAR AND ADRENAL FUNCTION

Another problem associated with sugar is particularly relevant to the subject of stress. Sugar is yet another substance that increases adrenaline release. Taken in excessive amounts, sugar could therefore be implicated in many of the side-effects associated with an overabundance of adrenaline. If this high intake were to continue for a prolonged period, it could lead to adrenal weakness and its symptoms, especially in overstressed individuals.

The over-consumption of sugar also may also lead to rebound hypoglycaemia. In this situation, the high intake of sugar ironically leads to low blood sugar due to an excessive level of insulin remaining in the blood after the consumed sugar has been metabolised. This scenario accounts, at least to an extent, for the 'crash' in energy levels often experienced a short while after the initial stimulating effect of sugar. The adrenaline release also wears off, leading to a drop in the level of certain body functions – and energy.

The possible risks of excessive sugar intake in stressed individuals is liable to be greatly increased by the consumption of caffeine, nicotine, and/or alcohol. Unfortunately, many people regularly consume both high levels of sugar and one or more of the other elements. Research has found that smokers tend to have a higher intake of caffeine, alcohol and sugar than non-smokers.

OTHER CONCERNS

Excessive sugar consumption is also associated with immune-system suppression and cardiovascular disease. This is especially important to note considering the risks that already exist due to chronic stress.

Salt

Salt is one of the more prominent sources of sodium in our diets. The minerals sodium and potassium play a major role in the effect that stress can have on the body (*see page 63*), particularly the cardiovascular system. If the fine balance between these two minerals is altered, certain problems may occur.

The links between salt and high blood pressure have been publicised to the extent that less salt is now added to food at the dinner table. The publicity did not, however, highlight the really important point of the research.

REDUCING SALT IS NOT ENOUGH

Only about one in five of us are 'salt sensitive' – those who are may be helped by reducing salt intake. What about the other 80 per cent? Research states is that it is the balance between sodium and potassium levels that really matters. We know that this is the case in the body, so why should the same principle not also apply to the diet? After all, our diet is the only source we have of both minerals.

The real problem with salt lies with food selection, and is not the fault of salt itself. The foods that would offer high potassium and proportionately low sodium content are vegetables and fruits. These are rather lacking in the typical Western diet, at least in comparison to the intake of processed foods, meat, dairy products, many junk foods, and table salt. (For a list of foods with a more appropriate potassium-to-sodium ratio, *see pages 65–6.*)

SALT AND STRESS

Release of the adrenal hormones during stress (especially aldosterone) leads to retention of sodium and loss of potassium. As a result, the balance between these minerals is greatly disrupted. When you add this to the typical problems with a dietary imbalance, the result is quite worrying. This is not only the case in the risk of high blood pressure, atherosclerosis and diagnosable diseases. Deficiencies in potassium inside the cells may also lead to problems such as muscle weakness, dizziness or confusion, nervous disorders and muscle cramp.

This is not to suggest that all sodium should be eliminated from the diet in favour of massive levels of potassium, as this also may produce an imbalance. It is just important to understand which way your diet is taking you, so that you can address the balance appropriately.

Meat

The consumption of meat should be moderate. Although such foods are unlikely to reduce one's stress tolerance greatly, if eaten several times a week they may increase some of the cardiovascular risks of chronic stress. This is particularly the case for beef and pork, and cured and processed meats, such as bacon, sausage and ham.

MEAT AND CARDIOVASCULAR HEALTH

The above types of meat contain higher quantities of saturated fats and cholesterol than is desirable. Diets high in these types of fats are associated with an increased risk of atherosclerosis. The cured and processed meats, besides containing these fats, also contain sodium in excess of the acceptable levels (this problem also applies to certain kinds of smoked fish, such as kippers and haddock). Much of these concerns can be eliminated, however, by balancing the diet with lots of fruit and vegetables.

Dairy Products

Many dairy products present problems very similar to those of meat. The sodium concerns, however, may be even worse. Saturated fat and cholesterol is almost always a worry when foods such as milk, cheese, cream, and butter are used, and lower-fat alternatives can be helpful in reducing this concern. It appears, however, that many standard margarines are actually more damaging to the cardiovascular system than butter due to their content of hydrogenated fats. In such cases, a little unsalted butter may be preferable.

Sodium-to-potassium ratios are also unfavourable in dairy products with respect to cardiovascular health. As with meat consumption, an increased intake of fresh fruits and vegetables is advisable if dairy products are consumed regularly.

POSITIVE FOODS

There are fortunately many foods that can actually provide a beneficial effect on stress tolerance. As a rule, the diet should not only limit the intake of the negative items discussed above, but should also include higher amounts of foods rich in anti-stress nutrients. Foods that may correct some of the associated health problems caused by the negative foods should also be increased.

Whole Grains
The food family of whole grains includes some of the most nutritionally rich and healthy foods. Some of the primary members include:

• wheat

- rice
- oats
- barley
- rye
- corn

These grains have many beneficial attributes relevant to an anti-stress programme and provide a source of complex carbohydrates (the sugars in complex carbohydrates are released gradually, without adversely affecting blood-sugar levels).

VITAMINS AND MINERALS

Whole grains contain many essential vitamins, minerals and other nutrients which are of great value in improving stress tolerance. They are particularly good sources of B-vitamins, including several necessary for the healthy functioning of the nervous system and adrenals. Whole grains are also a good source of other anti-stress nutrients such as zinc and magnesium. (Anti-stress nutrients will be discussed in more depth in Chapter Six.)

POTASSIUM:SODIUM RATIO

Whole grains also provide a helpful tool to rebalance dietary intake of potassium and sodium as there is a good ratio between the two minerals. They are also free of the other negative attributes often found in high-sodium foods (*see pages 65–6*).

FIBRE

An exceptional source of dietary fibre, whole grains improve intestinal health and regularity. The fibre contained in certain grains, such as oats, may reduce some of the concerns of a diet high in fat and cholesterol by speeding their removal from the intestines.

> **PLEASE NOTE:** The excellent nutritional value of whole grains, including the potassium:sodium ratio and fibre content, is dependent on the grain being 'whole'. Brown rice, for example, is preferable to white rice, and whole-wheat is preferable to foods made with white flour.

Beans and Other Legumes

This is another food family that provides high levels of nutrition, and is generally without negative attributes. Some of the most healthy and nutritionally suitable members of this category include:

- soybeans
- kidney beans
- broad beans
- lentils
- chickpeas

Like whole grains, the legumes are excellent sources of the anti-stress B-vitamins; many minerals, such as zinc, calcium and magnesium; dietary fibre (including the type that is of most benefit to the cardiovascular system), high protein, and complex carbohydrates. Legumes also have a good potassium:sodium ratio.

Fresh Fruits and Vegetables

Most people know that a healthy diet should contain lots of fresh fruits and vegetables. For sufferers of stress and its associated problems, this is especially so. These foods contain a favourable amount of essential vitamins and minerals. As each category has its own nutritional strengths, it is a good idea for the stressed individual to consume liberal quantities of both. These foods are also very good sources of dietary fibre.

One of the main benefits of the increased consumption of fruits and vegetables on stress tolerance stems from their potassium content. They provide perhaps the best method of correcting the imbalance produced by the typical 'Western' way of eating. As mentioned earlier, this is particularly important to the health of the cardiovascular system.

Potassium:sodium Ratio – Foods to Eat and to Avoid

Listed below is a selection of some of the best and worst foods in terms of high potassium to sodium ratios.

BEST
- bananas
- avocados

- oranges
- buckwheat
- rye
- whole-wheat
- soybeans
- haricot beans (dry)
- tomatoes
- plums
- asparagus
- corn
- apples
- strawberries
- potatoes

WORST

- bacon
- sausage
- butter (salted)
- cheese (in general)
- kippers
- white bread
- many condiments (e.g. ketchup)
- many processed breakfast cereals
- many packaged snack foods
- many canned foods

If any of the foods on the 'worst' list are eaten regularly, members of the 'best' list should also be eaten frequently to compensate. People suffering from stress must, however, be careful. The higher their stress levels and/or their risk of cardiovascular problems, the less they can afford to test their tolerance for the negative foods.

The basic guidelines in this chapter should help you to compensate, at least to an extent, for the effects of excessive stress levels in your life. If nothing else, it should help you to avoid making matters worse. In addition to their direct effect on stress tolerance and adrenal support, many of the nutrients contained in the positive foods are helpful in reducing risks to the cardiovascular system, the immune system, and literally every system of the body.

IMPORTANT: When one is under stress there is a tendency for one to consume more sugar, caffeine, nicotine and alcohol. Even if you stop consuming these substances, long-term ingestion in the past could have already taken its toll on the body. As a result, it is vital to take advantage of the foods that provide nutritional support and protection to the body, rather than just eliminating as many negative foods as you can manage.

CHAPTER 6

Natural Therapy for Stress Protection and Improved Stress Tolerance

No matter what the health problem, it is vital to assess every possible contributing factor. As it is unrealistic to avoid stress factors completely, the best approach for sufferers is to find out what may reduce the negative effects, or enhance their ability to handle the inevitable. Diet is an example of this. But what happens if it is not feasible to compensate adequately for the effect stress is having (or has already had) on the body through dietary changes alone? To coin a phrase, what you put into your body is bound to have a substantial bearing on what you get out of your body.

There are a few major reasons why diet alone may not be enough:

1 A more aggressive approach may be needed to reverse the damaging effects of long-term chronic stress on the body's 'stress network' (such as the adrenal glands and supply of hormones).

2 The stress may be far too severe to be compensated

for with changes in food alone.

3 It may be necessary to strengthen other areas of the body adversely affected by stress (such as the cardiovascular and immune systems). This often involves more than food changes alone.

4 Even the best diets often do not provide adequate nutrition to maintain damaged or over-worked body systems properly. Research is now suggesting that a good diet may not be enough to protect even healthy body systems from stress.

THE VALUE OF NUTRITIONAL SUPPLEMENTATION AND HERBAL MEDICINE

As there are limitations to the effectiveness of dietary changes alone, it is necessary to have an additional method of bolstering the body. Although a healthy diet does contain the nutrients needed to maintain body systems, quantities are the problem. It is not enough just to ingest the right nutrients – they must be taken in the amounts needed by the body.

To meet these levels through foods alone would mean eating quantities far in excess of what is realistic; and this is not taking into account the amount of nutrients which are destroyed through:

• cooking
• processing
• canning

- freezing
- lack of freshness
- soil-depletion

This is where the value of food supplementation becomes most evident. If you cannot get enough in your diet, then you must get it elsewhere. Fortunately, there are supplements to bridge the gap between what is eaten and what is really needed.

There are also times when people with health problems or challenges can benefit from herbal medicine. Stress is no exception. There are constituents in herbs that can offer protection, strengthening and/or stimulation to any conceivable function of the body.

A realistic and effective approach appears to be:

1 utilising the beneficial effects of dietary changes
2 supplementing the diet with nutrients where most appropriate
3 taking advantage of the relevant benefits the herbal kingdom has to offer.

In combination with various relaxation techniques, exercise, and psychological support if necessary, this approach can give sufferers one of the best chances of dealing with their stress. This chapter outlines the most appropriate nutritional and herbal methods of increasing stress tolerance and protection. All suggested methods are safe and natural, and based on research published in highly respected scientific and medical journals.

B-VITAMINS

The several different types of B-vitamin are known collectively as the vitamin B-complex. The more valuable food sources of the individual B-vitamins include whole grains (especially brown rice), liver, and brewer's yeast.

Each B-vitamin has its own effects on the body. Many relate to the function of the central nervous system and adrenal glands. The nervous system takes a beating under emotional/mental stress. Many B-vitamins either protect against nerve damage and/or exert a calming or nerve-relaxing effect. Such abilities are very important in reducing the long-term 'nervous exhaustion' often seen in over-stressed people. They may also succeed in 'taking the edge off' the more common stress symptoms, such as anxiety, irritability, tension and insomnia. There are many other symptoms and conditions associated with deficiencies in the B-vitamins listed below, but these are some of the ones more relevant to symptoms of stress and nervous disorders.

Pantothenic Acid (vitamin B$_5$)

Pantothenic acid, or vitamin B$_5$, is often called the 'anti-stress vitamin'. It is an 'essential' vitamin, which means that it is needed in order to sustain life, but that the body cannot create its own adequate supply without intake of the nutrient from the diet. Pantothenic acid serves many different purposes in the body, including energy production within body cells, but the most relevant function to stress is its effect on the adrenals.

THE ADRENALS

This nutrient is essential for the body's production of adrenal hormones. If the dietary intake is too low to compensate for the levels of such hormones used up during stress, then the hormone supply will be reduced (research has also suggested that this can lead to atrophy of the adrenal gland). Pantothenic acid is therefore of great value in reducing the risk of adrenal exhaustion from chronic stress.

PHYSICAL STRESS

Research of particular interest has revealed that pantothenic acid can have a protective effect against physical stress. This is based on the results of studies on both humans and animals which suggest that a higher than normal intake of pantothenic acid may greatly increase endurance under conditions of extreme physical stress.

SOURCES

Pantothenic acid is found in many foods. Rich sources include:

- beans and other legumes
- liver
- whole grains (e.g. brown rice, whole-wheat)
- tomatoes

In cases of chronic stress, it would be unrealistic to try and obtain therapeutic amounts of vitamin B$_5$ without supplementation. Achieving a high intake of the vitamin through food should, however, be a major dietary priority.

DOSAGE

The amount of pantothenic acid required varies greatly from person to person, and is determined partly by the levels of stress being experienced. Fortunately, B$_5$ is virtually non-toxic, and thus offers more flexibility than might be expected (this is true for a wide variety of essential nutrients). A range of 100–200 milligrams (mg) per day is probably acceptable for milder forms of chronic stress, while 200–1,000 mg is often used when stress levels are more severe. The benefits of B$_5$ can also be applied to acute, but temporary, stress. In such cases, it might be appropriate to consider 500–1,000 mg per day.

Vitamin B$_6$ (pyridoxine)

This vitamin has two very important functions in relation to stress. Firstly, it is necessary for the production of adrenal hormones. When the levels of such hormones are depleted under stress, the requirements for B_6 increase. Secondly, B_6 is vital for a properly functioning nervous system. A deficiency in this essential vitamin, which is not at all unusual, is linked to neurological disorders, nervousness, and depression. Although these are general observations, such benefits have been particularly well documented in the case of premenstrual tension (PMT).

Vitamin B_{12} (cobalamin)

This vitamin is required for protection of nerve endings, so long-term deficiency can result in nerve damage. Inadequate intake has also been associated with irritability and depression. It is particularly difficult to obtain adequate quantities of Vitamin B_{12} in vegetarian, and especially vegan diets, so supplementation is even more valuable in such cases.

Vitamin B_1 (thiamine)

This nutrient plays a valuable role in proper nerve function. Some of the symptoms that can be caused by a deficiency of vitamin B_1 include irritability, anxiety, nervousness and depression.

Vitamin B_3 (niacin/niacinamide)

This essential vitamin can produce calming properties due to its activity in the brain. Deficiencies in vitamin B_3 are linked to irritability, insomnia, and depression. In higher doses, niacin may cause a harmless and temporary flushing, particularly when supplements are taken between meals and in levels in excess of 50–100 mg. Niacinamide (another form of vitamin B_3, is not associated with such flushing.

PABA (para-aminobenzoic acid)
Deficiencies in PABA can lead to irritability and depression.

Biotin
A deficiency in biotin may cause insomnia and depression.

Folic acid
Folic acid deficiency can cause insomnia and apathy.

Vitamin B-Complex
As with pantothenic acid, it is unrealistic to expect to achieve therapeutic levels of the other important B-vitamins from daily food intake alone. Therapeutic amounts can, however, be obtained through supplementation with vitamin B-complex (which also can be found in multiple vitamin/mineral preparations). The typical B-complex contains:

- B_1 (thiamine)
- B_2 (riboflavin)
- B_6 (pyridoxine)
- B_{12} (cobalamin)

- biotin
- choline
- folic acid
- inositol
- niacinamide or niacin (B_3)
- pantothenic acid (B_5)
- PABA (para-aminobenzoic acid)

DOSAGE

Recommended dosages for each of the B-vitamins depend on individual needs. In addition to the separate requirements for pantothenic acid, a B-complex supplement containing approximately 50–100 mg. of most of the B-vitamins may provide very helpful assistance to the body's fight against stress. Some multiple vitamin/mineral formulas will contain the B-complex vitamins within this potency range. In a B-complex, some of the B-vitamins (B_{12}, biotin and folic acid) are found in microgram (mcg) rather than milligram (mg) doses.

VITAMIN C

Also known as ascorbic acid, vitamin C is one of the best-known nutrients, and one of the most vital during stress.

Vitamin C is found in very large quantities in the adrenal glands, but the research into why this is the case is fairly confusing. A couple of strong observations have, however, been made. Firstly, levels of vitamin C have been shown to be significantly reduced when one is under stress. This suggests that people suffering from stress need higher intakes of vitamin C in order to maintain necessary levels. Secondly, one particular study showed that people who received high doses of vitamin C excreted more adrenaline under stress than those with a low intake. This suggests that vitamin C plays a role in adrenaline activity under stress. As adrenaline is needed for the body's initial tolerance and adjustment for stress, increased vitamin C may enhance 'preparedness' for stress. Aside from the probable reduction in stress tolerance, inadequate intake of this essential nutrient would also increase the likelihood of other stress-related problems.

Immunity

Research shows that vitamin C stimulates the immune system. It speeds up the production of interferon and the activity of white blood cells and antibodies. For people suffering from stress, vitamin C is particularly important. This is because the activity of the immune system is weakened by the adrenal hormones secreted during stress.

Cardiovascular Disease

Cardiovascular disorders, such as atherosclerosis and high blood pressure, can be linked to stress (*see pages 23–8*). The activity of vitamin C in the body may significantly reduce such concerns in addition to improving stress tolerance in general.

Vitamin C has a strengthening effect on the walls of the blood vessels, and it has been suggested that it may reduce the risk of injury to the arterial wall. Such an injury may lead to the development of atherosclerosis in the first place.

The build-up of arterial plaque seen in atherosclerosis is partially made of cholesterol deposits (*see page 27*). Vitamin C reduces the deposition of fat and cholesterol in general, and thus would likely reduce the risk of plaque development.

SOURCES

Not only citrus fruits, but fresh fruits in general provide good quantities of vitamin C. In vegetables, it is most abundant in broccoli and cauliflower. To get the most out of fruits and vegetables, they should be as fresh as possible. Cooking destroys quite a bit of the vitamin C as well as other important vitamins.

Supplements of vitamin C are quite popular during the cold season, but they may also come in handy for stressed individuals who want a more practical way of ingesting therapeutic amounts.

Dosage

Vitamin C has many vital functions. One of its major roles is in the production of collagen, the most abundant protein in the body, which is prominent in connective tissue. With this and all its other uses in mind, the requirement for vitamin C is important regardless of stress. A lack of vitamin C has been linked to irritability, depression, weakened immunity, cardiovascular dysfunction, and many other problems.

Dosages of vitamin C depend on individual needs, but a realistic daily amount to aid in protection from chronic stress might be 500–1,500 mg. As vitamin C is excreted rather quickly from the body even under normal circumstances, it is preferable for larger amounts to be divided over the day rather than all used at once.

ZINC

The essential mineral zinc is vital to many bodily functions, and has both a direct and an indirect role in stress. It affects stress tolerance in a direct manner because it is necessary for the production of adrenal hormones. As with pantothenic acid, vitamin B_6 and others, zinc becomes depleted, or is used up more quickly, during stress. It is therefore very important to ensure that the levels are replenished. Unfortunately, even a diet rich in zinc may be inadequate to deal with chronic stress and many other factors.

The Immune System

Zinc is also a primary nutrient in the activity of the immune system. Many of the immune functions which are impaired by stress can be stimulated by zinc. Its major benefits to the immune system are:

1 protecting against shrinkage of the thymus gland
2 increasing the number and activity of T-cells (immune-stimulating white blood cells from the thymus gland)
3 increasing antibody function
4 maintaining adequate supply of thymus hormones

Inadequate levels of zinc are linked to many conditions and symptoms relevant to stress, such as irritability, depression, impotence and weak immunity. It is therefore vital for people suffering from chronic stress to have an adequate intake of zinc.

Sources

Common foods rich in zinc include whole grains (e.g. brown rice), beans, seeds (especially pumpkin and sesame), nuts and liver. Zinc supplements come in many forms, and are very practical for ensuring adequate levels. It is advisable, however, to use a form that offers better absorption of the zinc into the body's cells, such as zinc picolinate, zinc amino acid chelate or zinc citrate.

Dosage

As zinc is involved in so many actions in human biochemistry, dosage requirements are difficult to determine, but for stressed individuals, somewhere in the range of 15–30 mg per day should be appropriate. Bear in mind that there may be a tendency for zinc to be depleted by certain factors, including alcohol intake, smoking, excessive sugar intake, infections and injuries.

Although there are times when higher amounts of zinc may be used to correct a particular health problem, it is suggested that the daily dosage should not exceed around 100 mg for long periods, as this may actually *suppress* immunity.

MAGNESIUM

Although most well known for its vital role in bone health (with calcium), the mineral magnesium also has many different actions, some which are very relevant to stress.

Adrenal Hormones

As with pantothenic acid, zinc and vitamins B6 and C, magnesium is involved in the manufacture and activity of adrenal hormones, and therefore helps reduce the risk of adrenal exhaustion from chronic stress.

The Nervous System

Magnesium causes the 'relaxation' of nerves, a vital role in the nervous system. This is of great value in cases of chronic or acute stress when the nerves are in a constant state of excitability. Studies on the effects of magnesium showed that it had substantial benefits in reducing daytime anxiety as well as improving night-time sleep patterns. Magnesium also relaxes muscles, which may help reduce stress-induced muscle stiffness and tension.

Magnesium and Calcium

As well as co-operating in bone health, magnesium and calcium also work together for nerve function. Magnesium relaxes the nerve cells, and calcium stimulates them. A proper balance of the two minerals may therefore be very helpful in maintaining proper nerve activity during stress – allowing for better nerve response, but preventing it from becoming excessive. This same relationship applies to the action of muscle relaxation and muscle contraction.

Cardiovascular Disorders

One of the most promising areas of research into the benefits of magnesium has been in cardiovascular disease. Magnesium can reduce the risk of, or even correct, many aspects of heart and blood-vessel disorders. It improves the function of the heart muscle, and helps to regulate and strengthen heart contractions. At the same time it may help correct an irregular heartbeat and reduce the chance of coronary-artery spasm, a possible cause of heart attacks.

REDUCING BLOOD PRESSURE

Research has shown magnesium supplementation to be effective in reducing blood pressure in many cases. This is due to its effects on two other minerals: potassium and sodium. Potassium is needed in higher quantities inside the cells, while sodium should be found mostly in the fluid outside the cells. Magnesium is involved in keeping excessive sodium out of the cells, and retaining potassium inside the cells. The improper distribution of sodium inside the cells is a major contributor to high blood pressure, and is often the result of low magnesium levels.

For best results, magnesium may be combined with calcium, as increased calcium intake appears to increase the elimination of sodium through the urine.

REDUCING ATHEROSCLEROSIS DEVELOPMENT

Magnesium supplementation has been found to reduce the tendency for blood to clot excessively, a major factor in the development of atherosclerosis (*see pages 27–8*). Reducing the risk of high blood pressure through magnesium intake may also decrease a tendency for atherosclerosis, as extreme blood pressure may increase the likelihood injury to the arterial wall and a subsequent build-up of plaque (*see page 28*).

CONTROLLING ALDOSTERONE

The stress-induced hormone aldosterone contributes significantly to cardiovascular risks. It causes retention of sodium and excretion of potassium, helping to maintain high blood pressure during the stress response. Research has shown that low magnesium levels lead to greater aldosterone levels.

Sources

Some of the best food sources of magnesium include whole grains (e.g. whole wheat, millet, rye, brown rice), nuts, seaweed, fresh green vegetables and beans. As with many nutrients, magnesium is easily lost when foods are processed or cooked. Calcium, which works in harmony with magnesium, is found in dairy products, nuts, seeds, beans, seaweed and many vegetables.

In order to ensure adequate intake, supplementation of magnesium is becoming more popular; in many cases it may be necessary in order to achieve therapeutic levels. There are many forms of magnesium supplements, and some are easier to absorb than others. (This is an important issue with minerals, as impaired absorption makes them less effective.) The most suitable forms of magnesium include magnesium citrate, magnesium amino acid chelate and magnesium aspartate. Magnesium supplements that also contain calcium may be useful and are often found in the approximate proportions listed below.

Dosage

Magnesium deficiency has been linked with irritability, anxiety, depression, cardiovascular dysfunction, insomnia, nervousness, muscle spasms, and other problems. Calcium deficiency is associated with nervousness, insomnia, irritability, depression and cardiovascular dysfunction. As magnesium co-operates with calcium to regulate many such actions on the nerves and muscles, and as both may reduce high blood pressure, it is often suggested that the two minerals are supplemented in tandem.

As with the other nutrients, adequate dosage depends on individual requirements, but 400–500 mg of magnesium and 800–1,000 mg of calcium may be suitable. Bear in mind that alcohol, stress, diuretics, and use of oral contraceptives can drain the body of magnesium, thus increasing the intake requirement.

POTASSIUM

Potassium is one of the most important nutrients in relation to chronic stress (*see page 63*). As well as maintaining sodium and fluid balance, it is involved in the proper functioning of almost every cell in the body, with an particular affinity for the nerves, muscles and especially the heart. Inadequate potassium levels may lead to insomnia, nervousness and depression.

Sources

Potassium is easier to obtain from foods than many other nutrients, provided that the proper foods are consumed. Some of the richer sources of dietary potassium include fresh fruits (e.g. bananas, oranges, apples), avocados, buckwheat, beans and whole grains (*see also list on pages 65–6*).Bear in mind that it is important not just to increase potassium intake, but to also achieve a more beneficial potassium:sodium ratio.

Supplementation may be used if, for whatever reason, the potassium: sodium ratio is not balanced through dietary measures. Although unusual with nutrient supplementation, potassium supplements do not typically contain large amounts of potassium compared to food intake*. As a result, one should only look to use potassium supplements as an adjunct to dietary change.

Dosage

As stress-induced adrenal hormones, especially aldosterone, cause substantial potassium loss, the intake

---

* As with all mineral supplements (e.g. zinc, magnesium, calcium), the quantity of actual potassium in a supplement is based on what is known as the elemental mineral content. (Minerals are not found by themselves in supplements; they are bonded or attached to other substances, e.g. zinc picolinate and magnesium citrate. The elemental mineral content refers to the potency of the mineral itself.)

must be adequate to compensate. Potassium loss can also be caused by diarrhoea, the use of diuretics (pills that relieve fluid retention), and medical use of corticosteroids (e.g. cortisone). In spite of the concern over exercise-induced potassium loss (through sweat), very large amounts are not likely to be lost in this manner.

The current point of view on reasonable adult intake levels of potassium points to approximately 2,000–6,000 mg per day. While a one-to-one ratio of potassium to sodium would be a vast improvement in the current intake of many people, it is suggested that sodium intake should probably be no more than around 1,000–3,000 mg per day.

KOREAN AND SIBERIAN GINSENG

On of the most well-known members of the herbal kingdom, ginseng comes in different varieties, and is grown mostly in Korea, China and the United States. One of the most potent and highly researched types is Korean ginseng. Another plant known as ginseng, even though it belongs to a different family of herbs, is *Eleutherococcus senticosus*, or Siberian Ginseng. This has also undergone research which has shown some of its most important values.

Many different claims have been made about these plants, creating a great deal of controversy as to what ginseng really does. Fortunately, research has now been published which validates at least some of the claims. Apart from the more common beliefs about ginseng being an energy tonic, and so on, the research points to the herb's capabilities in protecting against stress.

Adaptogenic Effect

Both Korean and Siberian ginseng belong to a category of substances called adaptogens. The term refers to a substance which offers 'non-specific resistance' – or more simply put, increases the body's ability to tolerate various stressors (e.g. mental, physical, and environ-mental). Research suggests that this benefit is to a great extent derived from a stabilising action on the adrenal glands. Considering the role of the adrenals in stress, this is not surprising.

The Adrenals

The activity of ginseng on the adrenal glands has a very wide scope. It:

1 increases the blood levels of certain adrenal hormones
2 increases blood levels of ACTH (pituitary hormone which regulates release of adrenal corticosteroid activity)
3 protects against shrinkage of adrenal glands caused by stress

For the over-stressed individual, the third point listed

above is one of the most valuable functions of ginseng. Stress, especially the chronic variety, can cause shrinkage of the adrenal glands. This ultimately weakens the glands, and thus the body's ability to deal with stress as it was intended. By virtue of its protection against this phenomenon, ginseng increases stress tolerance and stress protection.

Active Constituents

The adaptogenic constituents of ginseng are known as 'ginsenosides'. Different ginsenosides are found in ginseng, and they have a variety of effects on the body. It is thought that the adaptogenic activity of species such as Panax ginseng (Korean or Chinese ginseng) is somewhat more potent than that of Siberian.

Specific ginsenosides are also found to reduce fatigue and improve the metabolism of fatty acids into energy. Such agents in Siberian ginseng have shown the ability to lower blood sugar when it becomes elevated by stress-induced corticosteroid release. Paradoxically, blood sugar that drops too low may become normalised by Siberian ginseng.

Safety

The different forms of ginseng appear to be safe to ingest, and research suggests that their toxicity is very low. Although adverse symptoms are generally very rare, nervousness, irritability, and hypertension are examples of reported side-effects in some individuals.

For this reason, it may be a good idea to move into ginseng supplementation gradually so that a more desirable level can be more easily achieved.

> **PLEASE NOTE:** Ginseng appears to contain small amounts of oestrogen. Women suffering from fibrocystic breast disease may find that excessive oestrogen causes breast pain and tenderness, and should therefore avoid ginseng.

Dosage

In spite of the rare exceptions, ginseng has much to offer to many over-stressed people. As one might expect, an effective dosage of ginseng will vary. This is not only the case from person to person, but it also depends on an individual's needs at any particular time. Dosage levels may also vary between different types. In spite of this rather confusing picture, 1,000– 2,000 mg of Korean ginseng or 1,000–3,000 mg of Siberian Ginseng may be appropriate for many. People who do not tolerate Korean ginseng, for whatever reason, may be able to use Siberian ginseng, although this is not always the case.

DIGESTIVE ENZYMES

The stress response has a tendency to inhibit severely the activity of certain body systems, including the digestive system, in favour of those most required for dealing with the stress (*see page 13*).

The digestive system is needed in order to supply the body with the nutrients required in order to live. If this process is impaired in any way, the body will naturally suffer the effects of under-nutrition. In other words, even if you eat plenty of food, the body cannot benefit from it until it is digested into its most basic components. Stress will impair this process, leading to other symptoms of digestive dysfunction including:

- indigestion
- gas
- abdominal bloating
- heartburn
- constipation and/or diarrhoea

Digestion is carried out by many different chemicals in the body known as digestive enzymes. The replacement of such enzymes after eating through supplementation may be helpful for relieving the symptoms and other consequences associated with improper digestion. Most, but not all, are secreted in the stomach, and from the pancreas into the first portion of the small intestine (duodenum). These main enzymes are:

STOMACH

- hydrochloric acid (digests proteins)

DUODENUM

- proteases (digests proteins)

- amylase (digests carbohydrates)
- lipase (digests fats)

Dosage

The appropriate dosage of digestive enzymes is based on the quantity of food intake, the types of food being consumed, the level of stress, and other factors. For people who are regularly over-stressed, it may be of value to use a digestive enzyme combination containing at least hydrochloric acid (e.g. betaine hydrochloride) and pancreatin (includes the three types of pancreatic enzymes). Such a formula should typically be used during or immediately after major meals.

IMPORTANT: Do *not* use formulas containing hydrochloric acid if you have a peptic ulcer.

Treatment Programme

The above supplements represent some of the most heavily researched, useful, and safe methods of increasing stress tolerance and protection. The following information represents a hypothetical programme which outlines the dietary changes and supplement recommendations which may be appropriate for a more successful anti-stress plan.

It is important to consult a qualified medical health practitioner before beginning this or any other health programme. Pregnant or lactating women, as well as children, should be particularly aware of the necessity for medical advice. This information is hypothetical and is *not* intended to be prescriptive in nature.

Avoid or reduce intake of:

- caffeine
- alcohol
- tobacco
- refined sugar
- salt (in excess)
- cured or processed meats (e.g. bacon, sausage, ham)
- processed food and junk-food snacks

(See pages 50–62 for further foods to avoid.)

Hypothetical recommendations (adult dosages):

- vitamin B-complex (50 mg, 1–2 times daily after food)
- pantothenic acid (vitamin B_5) (100–500 mg, 1–2 times daily after food)
- vitamin C (500 mg, 1–3 times daily)
- zinc (picolinate, amino acid chelate or citrate) (15–30 mg, once daily)
- calcium and magnesium (as citrate) (800–1,000 mg, 400–500 mg daily)
- Korean ginseng (1,000–2,000 mg daily) *or* Siberian ginseng (1,000–3,000 mg daily)

Optional:

- potassium (e.g. aspartate, gluconate) (100–150 mg daily in addition to dietary potassium intake)
- digestive enzyme combination (as directed on label during or immediately after major meals, do not take without doctor's advice if suffering with a peptic ulcer)

BIBLIOGRAPHY

Abou-Saleh, M. and Coppen, A. *Journal of Psychiatric Research*, 20, 2, 1986, pp. 91–101.

Abraham, G. *Problems in Obstetric and Gynecology*, 3, 12, 1980, pp. 1–39.

Abraham, G. *Journal of Reproductive Medicine*, 28, 7, 1983, pp. 446–64.

Alberti, K. and Nattrass, M. *Lancet*, 2, 1977, pp. 25–9.

Arnesen, E. *et al. British Medical Journal*, 288, 1984, p. 1,960.

Bennet, A. *et al. Lancet*, i, 1970, pp. 1,011–14.

Bensky, D. and Gamble, A. *Chinese Herbal Medicine: Materia Medica*, Eastland Press, 1986, pp. 236, 452–4.

Bland, J. *et al. Medical Applications of Clinical Nutrition*, Keats, 1983, pp. 184, 211.

Bolton, S. and Null, G. *Journal of Orthomolecular Psychiatry*, 10, 1981, pp. 210–11.

Bombardelli, E *et al. Proceedings of the Third International Ginseng Symposium*, 1980, pp. 9–16.

Brekhman, I. and Dardymov, I. *Lloydia*, 32, 1969, pp. 46–51.

Buist, R. *International Clinical Nutrition Review*, 5, 1985, pp. 1–4.

Carney, M. *et al. British Journal of Psychiatry*, 141, 1982, pp. 271–2.

Crammer, J. *Psychol. Med.*, 7, 1977, pp. 557–60.

D'Angelo, L. *et al, Journal of Ethnopharmacology*, 16, 1986, pp. 15–22.

Friedman, M. *American Heart Journal*, 97, 1979, p. 114.

Fulder, S. *American Journal of Chinese Medicine*, 9, 1981, pp. 112–18.

Gianella, R. *et al. Annals of Internal Medicine*, 78, 1973, pp. 271–6.

Griffin, J. and Ojeda, S. *Textbook of Endocrine Physiology*, OUP, 1992.

Hodges, R. and Rebello, T.

'Carbohydrates and blood pressure', *Annals of Internal Medicine*, 98, 1983, pp. 838–41.

Holmes, T. and Rahe, R. *Journal of Psychosomatic Research*, 11, 1967, pp. 213–18.

Innerfield, I. *Enzymes in Clinical Medicine*, McGraw Hill, New York, 1960.

Kawasaki, T. *et al. American Journal of Medicine*, 64, 1978, pp. 193–8.

Khaw, K. and Thom, S. *Lancet*, 2, 1982, pp. 1,127–9.

Kirshbaum, A. *et al. Journal of the American Medical Association*, 203, 1968, pp. 113–16.

Liebman, B. *Nutrition Action*, Nov. 1981, p. 9.

McCarron, D. and Morris, C. *Annals of Internal Medicine*, 102, 1985, pp. 825–31.

Miller, G. *Journal Nat. Med. Assoc.*, 76, 1, 1984, pp. 47–52.

Mohler, H. *et al. Nature*, 278, 1979, pp. 563–5.

Morris, J. and Chave, S. *Lancet*, 6 Dec., 1980, p. 1,207.

Murray, M. and Pizzorno, J. *Encyclopaedia of Natural Medicine*, Macdonald, 1990.

Nutrition Foundation, *Present Knowledge in Nutrition*, fifth edition, 1984.

Powers, H. *Academics and Therapeutics*, 9, 1973, p. 203.

Prasad, A. *et al. Annals of Internal Medicine*, 89, 1978, p. 483.

Rabkin, J. and Stuening, E. *Science*, 191, 1976, p. 1,013.

Rainey, J. *et al. Psychopharmacology Bulletin*, 20, 1, 1984, p. 45–9.

Riley, V. *Science*, 189, 1975, p. 465.

Sakai, Y. and Stone, R. *International Journal of Epidemiology*, 6, 1977, p. 7.

Scauff, C. *et al. Human Physiology*, Times Mirror/Mosby College, St Louis, Mo., 1990.

Schorah, C. *et al, Human Nutrition: Clinical Nutrition*, 37, 1983, pp. 447–52.

Seelig, M. and Heegtveit, H. *American Journal of Clinical Nutrition*, 27, 1974, pp. 59–79.

Selye, H. *The General Adaptation Syndrome*, Bantam, New York, 1972.

Selye, H. *Stress in Health and Disease*, Butterworths, 1976.

Sydenstricker, V. *et al. Journal of the American Medical Association*, 118, 1940, pp. 1,199–200.

Wetterberg, L. and Unden, F. *Lancet*, 10 July 1982, p. 100.

Willer, J. and Cambier, J. *Science*, 212, 1982, p. 689.

Zucker, D. *et al. Biol. Psychiat.*, 16, 1981, pp. 197–205.